SURVIVING HASHIMOTO'S

A Guide to Thriving with Autoimmune Thyroid Disease

By David Lefkon and Artificial Intelligence

TABLE OF CONTENTS

CHAPTER 1: INTRODUCTION TO HASHIMOTO'S 1

Understanding Hashimoto's Thyroiditis 2
The Autoimmune Response 3
Symptoms of Hashimoto's 4
Diagnosing Hashimoto's 5
Importance of Early Diagnosis 7
Overview of Treatment and Management 8

CHAPTER 2: SYMPTOMS AND IMPACT ON DAILY LIFE 10

Understanding the Symptoms of Hashimoto's 11
Common Symptoms 12
Less Common Symptoms 13
Impact on Daily Life 14
Work and Productivity 15
Social Life and Relationships 16
Mental Health and Well-Being 17
Physical Health 18

CHAPTER 3: DIAGNOSING HASHIMOTO'S THYROIDITIS 20

The Path to Diagnosis..21
Initial Consultation..22
Diagnostic Tests 23
Challenges in Diagnosis 24
Importance of Early Diagnosis 25
Working with Healthcare Providers 26

CHAPTER 4: TREATMENT AND MANAGEMENT OPTIONS 28

Overview of Treatment 29
Hormone Replacement Therapy 30
Dosage and Monitoring 31
Side Effects and Interactions 32
Additional Medications and Treatments 33
Lifestyle Changes..34
Alternative and Complementary Therapies 35
Supportive Care and Coping Strategies 36

CHAPTER 5: NAVIGATING LIFE WITH HASHIMOTO'S 38

The Emotional Impact of Hashimoto's 39
Building a Support System 40
Coping Strategies 41
Managing Work and Career 42

Navigating Relationships 43
Parenthood and Family Planning 44

CHAPTER 6: NUTRITION AND DIET FOR HASHIMOTO'S 46

The Role of Nutrition in Managing Hashimoto's 47
Key Nutrients for Thyroid Health 48
Foods to Include 49
Foods to Limit or Avoid 50
Dietary Approaches 51
Meal Planning and Preparation 52
Supplements and Considerations 53

CHAPTER 7: EXERCISE AND PHYSICAL ACTIVITY WITH HASHIMOTO'S 55

The Importance of Physical Activity 56
Benefits of Exercise 57
Types of Exercise 58
Creating an Exercise Plan 59
Managing Exercise-Induced Fatigue 60
Safety Considerations 61

CHAPTER 8: STRESS MANAGEMENT AND MENTAL HEALTH 63

The Connection Between Stress and Hashimoto's 64

Understanding the Effects of Stress 64
Effective Stress Management Techniques 65
Emotional Well-Being and Self-Care 66
Sleep and Stress Management 67
Seeking Support 68

CHAPTER 9: MEDICATION AND TREATMENT OPTIONS 70

Understanding Medication and Treatment 71
Thyroid Hormone Replacement Therapy 72
Finding the Right Dosage 73
Additional Medications and Supplements 74
Complementary and Alternative Treatments 75
Working with Your Healthcare Provider 76

CHAPTER 10: LIFESTYLE ADJUSTMENTS FOR LIVING WITH HASHIMOTO'S 78

Balancing Work and Rest 80
Staying Active 81
Managing Weight and Nutrition 82
Stress Management and Mental Health 83
Sleep Hygiene 84
Social and Emotional Support 85
Environmental Considerations 86
Monitoring and Regular Check-Ups 87

CHAPTER 11: BUILDING A SUPPORT NETWORK 89

The Importance of a Support Network 91
Building Your Support Network 92
Types of Support Groups 93
Nurturing Relationships with Loved Ones 94
Seeking Professional Support 95

CHAPTER 12: LONG-TERM MANAGEMENT AND MONITORING 97

The Importance of Long-Term Management 99
Adjusting Medication and Treatment 101
Preventing Complications 103
Building a Support Network 104

CHAPTER 13: COPING WITH HASHIMOTO'S AND DAILY LIFE 106

Navigating Daily Activities 108
Work-Life Balance 109
Coping with Fatigue 110
Emotional Well-being 111
Managing Relationships 112
Overcoming Brain Fog 113
Diet and Nutrition 114

CHAPTER 14: EXPLORING COMPLEMENTARY AND ALTERNATIVE THERAPIES 116

Understanding Complementary and Alternative Therapies 118
Acupuncture 119
Herbal Medicine 120
Dietary Supplements 121
Mind-Body Practices 122
Massage Therapy 123
Chiropractic Care 124
Aromatherapy 125

CHAPTER 15: COPING WITH SETBACKS AND FLARE-UPS 127

Understanding Setbacks and Flare-Ups 129
Coping Strategies for Setbacks and Flare-Ups 130
Managing Emotional Impact 131
Adjusting Treatment Plans 132
Preventing Future Setbacks 133
Building Resilience 134

CHAPTER 16: NAVIGATING RELATIONSHIPS AND SOCIAL LIFE 136

Communicating with Loved Ones 138
Managing Social Engagements 139
Addressing Relationship Challenges 140

Building a Support Network 141
Navigating Work Relationships 142
Balancing Personal and Social Life 143
Setting Realistic Expectations 144

CHAPTER 17: FAMILY PLANNING AND PREGNANCY WITH HASHIMOTO'S 146

Preconception Planning 148
Managing Pregnancy with Hashimoto's 149
Supporting a Healthy Pregnancy 150
Preparing for Childbirth 151
Postpartum Considerations 152

CHAPTER 18: TRAVEL AND ADVENTURE WITH HASHIMOTO'S 154

Planning Your Trip 156
Packing Essentials 157
Staying Healthy While Traveling 158
Adapting to New Environments 159
Navigating Travel Challenges 160
Embracing Adventure Safely 161

APPENDIX 163

A: Glossary of Terms 164
B: Recommended Reading and Resources 167

C: Sample Food Diary 169
D: Sample Medication Log 170
E: Frequently Asked Questions 171
F: Contact Information for Emergency Situations 173
G: Sample Blood Test Results and Interpretation 174
I: International Travel Considerations 176

DISCLAIMER 176

CHAPTER 1: INTRODUCTION TO HASHIMOTO'S

UNDERSTANDING HASHIMOTO'S THYROIDITIS

Hashimoto's thyroiditis, also known simply as Hashimoto's, is an autoimmune condition in which the immune system mistakenly attacks the thyroid gland. The thyroid gland is a small, butterfly-shaped organ located in the neck, just below the Adam's apple. It plays a vital role in regulating metabolism, energy levels, and many other bodily functions by producing essential hormones: thyroxine (T4) and triiodothyronine (T3).

In Hashimoto's, the immune system creates antibodies that target the thyroid gland as if it were a foreign invader. This autoimmune response leads to chronic inflammation and potential damage to the thyroid, resulting in a gradual decline in its function over time. As the thyroid gland loses its ability to produce adequate hormones, the body experiences various symptoms of hypothyroidism (underactive thyroid).

THE AUTOIMMUNE RESPONSE

Hashimoto's is an autoimmune disorder, which means the immune system attacks healthy tissue instead of harmful pathogens. In this case, the immune system produces antibodies, particularly thyroid peroxidase antibodies (TPOAb) and thyroglobulin antibodies (TgAb), that target the thyroid gland. This leads to chronic inflammation, reduced hormone production, and possible enlargement of the gland (goiter).

Autoimmune conditions like Hashimoto's are complex, and the exact cause is not entirely understood. However, genetic factors, environmental triggers, and other autoimmune disorders may contribute to the development of Hashimoto's.

SYMPTOMS OF HASHIMOTO'S

The symptoms of Hashimoto's can vary widely depending on the severity of the condition and how much the thyroid gland's function is compromised. Symptoms may develop gradually over time and may include:

- Fatigue: Persistent tiredness and lack of energy, even after rest.
- Weight Gain: Unexplained weight gain or difficulty losing weight.
- Sensitivity to Cold: Feeling unusually cold in normal temperatures.
- Dry Skin and Brittle Hair: Changes in skin texture and hair quality.
- Muscle Aches and Joint Pain: Persistent discomfort or pain in muscles and joints.
- Mood Changes: Depression, irritability, or anxiety.
- Irregular Menstrual Cycles: Changes in menstrual patterns, including heavy or irregular periods.
- Goiter: An enlarged thyroid gland, often noticeable as a swelling in the neck.
- Cognitive Impairment: Difficulty concentrating, memory issues, or brain fog.
- Constipation: Slower digestive processes can lead to constipation.

Symptoms can vary in intensity and frequency, often overlapping with other conditions, which can make diagnosis challenging.

DIAGNOSING HASHIMOTO'S

The diagnosis of Hashimoto's thyroiditis involves a comprehensive assessment that includes a review of medical history, physical examination, and specific blood tests to assess thyroid function and identify autoimmune markers:

- Thyroid-Stimulating Hormone (TSH): TSH is produced by the pituitary gland and stimulates the thyroid gland to produce T4 and T3 hormones. Elevated TSH levels can indicate hypothyroidism.

- Free T4 and T3: These blood tests measure the levels of the active thyroid hormones, thyroxine (T4) and triiodothyronine (T3). Low levels suggest an underactive thyroid.

- Thyroid Peroxidase Antibodies (TPOAb): This blood test measures the presence of antibodies against thyroid peroxidase, an enzyme involved in hormone production. High levels indicate an autoimmune response against the thyroid gland.

- Thyroglobulin Antibodies (TgAb): This test measures antibodies against thyroglobulin, a protein involved in thyroid hormone production. Elevated levels suggest autoimmune activity.

An ultrasound of the thyroid gland may also be performed to assess its size and structure, as well as to identify any nodules or other abnormalities.

IMPORTANCE OF EARLY DIAGNOSIS

Early diagnosis of Hashimoto's thyroiditis is essential for effective management and prevention of further thyroid damage. By identifying the condition in its early stages, treatment can begin sooner, reducing the risk of complications and improving overall quality of life.

Left untreated, Hashimoto's can lead to more severe hypothyroidism, causing worsening symptoms and potentially serious health issues such as heart problems, infertility, and depression. Additionally, an enlarged thyroid gland (goiter) can cause discomfort and difficulty swallowing.

OVERVIEW OF TREATMENT AND MANAGEMENT

Treatment for Hashimoto's typically involves hormone replacement therapy to restore thyroid hormone levels to a healthy range. The most common medication prescribed is levothyroxine, a synthetic form of T4. Proper dosage and regular monitoring of hormone levels are crucial for managing the condition effectively.

In addition to medication, other treatments and lifestyle changes may be recommended:

- Nutrition and Diet: A balanced diet that includes essential nutrients such as iodine, selenium, and zinc can support thyroid function. Avoiding foods that interfere with thyroid hormone absorption may also be beneficial.

- Exercise: Regular physical activity can help manage weight, boost energy levels, and improve mood.

- Stress Management: Chronic stress can exacerbate symptoms. Techniques such as mindfulness, meditation, or yoga can help manage stress.

- Adequate Sleep: Prioritizing quality sleep is important for overall health and well-being.

By incorporating these treatments and lifestyle adjustments, individuals with Hashimoto's can better manage their condition and improve their quality of life.

This chapter provides a comprehensive overview of Hashimoto's thyroiditis, including its nature, symptoms, diagnosis, and treatment options. The following chapters will delve deeper into specific aspects of managing the condition and share personal experiences and strategies to help you thrive while living with Hashimoto's.

CHAPTER 2: SYMPTOMS AND IMPACT ON DAILY LIFE

UNDERSTANDING THE SYMPTOMS OF HASHIMOTO'S

Hashimoto's thyroiditis manifests in various symptoms that can significantly affect daily life and overall well-being. The severity and combination of symptoms vary from person to person depending on the stage and extent of thyroid dysfunction. While some symptoms may appear early on, others may develop gradually over time.

COMMON SYMPTOMS

- Fatigue: Persistent and overwhelming tiredness is one of the most common symptoms. Even with adequate rest and sleep, individuals may feel depleted of energy.
- Weight Gain: Unexplained weight gain and difficulty losing weight can be frustrating. This occurs due to a slowed metabolism caused by hypothyroidism.
- Cold Sensitivity: Individuals may feel cold even in normal temperatures, and it can be challenging to stay warm.
- Dry Skin and Brittle Hair: The skin may become dry, flaky, and irritated, while hair may become brittle and prone to breakage.
- Muscle Aches and Joint Pain: Aching muscles and joint stiffness are frequent complaints, which can affect mobility and physical comfort.
- Mood Changes: Depression, irritability, anxiety, and mood swings are common due to hormonal imbalances and may impact relationships and daily interactions.
- Irregular Menstrual Cycles: For women, menstrual cycles may become heavy, light, or irregular due to disrupted hormone levels.
- Cognitive Impairment: Brain fog, difficulty concentrating, and memory problems can interfere with daily activities and work.
- Constipation: A slowed digestive system can lead to infrequent bowel movements and discomfort.
- Goiter: An enlarged thyroid gland (goiter) can cause a visible lump in the neck and may lead to difficulty swallowing or breathing.

LESS COMMON SYMPTOMS

- High Cholesterol: Hypothyroidism can lead to elevated cholesterol levels, increasing the risk of cardiovascular issues.

- Hoarseness: Changes in the voice, such as hoarseness or difficulty speaking, may occur due to inflammation of the thyroid.

- Carpal Tunnel Syndrome: Numbness, tingling, and pain in the hands and wrists can occur due to fluid retention and nerve compression.

IMPACT ON DAILY LIFE

The symptoms of Hashimoto's can have a significant impact on daily life. Here's how the condition can affect different aspects:

WORK AND PRODUCTIVITY

- Concentration and Focus: Cognitive impairment and brain fog can hinder concentration and productivity at work.

- Energy Levels: Fatigue may lead to decreased productivity and difficulty meeting work demands.

- Communication: Mood changes and hoarseness can affect communication and interpersonal relationships in the workplace.

SOCIAL LIFE AND RELATIONSHIPS

- Mood Changes: Irritability and mood swings can strain relationships with family and friends.
- Activity Levels: Fatigue and physical discomfort may limit participation in social activities.
- Self-Esteem: Changes in appearance and weight can impact self-esteem and confidence in social settings.

MENTAL HEALTH AND WELL-BEING

- Emotional Challenges: Anxiety and depression can take a toll on emotional well-being and may require support and treatment.

- Stress: Managing a chronic condition can be stressful, affecting overall mental health.

- Coping Strategies: Developing healthy coping strategies and seeking support can help manage emotional challenges.

PHYSICAL HEALTH

- Weight Management: Unexplained weight gain can lead to body image issues and may increase the risk of other health problems.

- Sleep Quality: Difficulty sleeping or maintaining sleep patterns can exacerbate fatigue and mood changes.

- Exercise: Muscle and joint pain may make physical activity more challenging, affecting overall health.

Conclusion

Understanding the range of symptoms and their impact on daily life is crucial for managing Hashimoto's thyroiditis effectively. Recognizing how the condition affects different aspects of life can guide individuals in making informed decisions about treatment and lifestyle adjustments. Seeking support and finding coping strategies can improve quality of life and help individuals thrive while living with Hashimoto's.

This chapter explores the symptoms and their impact on daily life for individuals with Hashimoto's. Subsequent chapters will delve into diagnosis and treatment options, as well as personal stories and coping strategies to navigate the journey with Hashimoto's.

CHAPTER 3: DIAGNOSING HASHIMOTO'S THYROIDITIS

THE PATH TO DIAGNOSIS

Diagnosing Hashimoto's thyroiditis can be a challenging and complex process. This is because the symptoms of Hashimoto's often overlap with other conditions, and some individuals may experience subtle or fluctuating symptoms. As a result, the journey to diagnosis may involve multiple medical visits, tests, and evaluations.

INITIAL CONSULTATION

The path to diagnosis usually begins with an initial consultation with a healthcare provider. During this appointment, the provider will gather a comprehensive medical history, including:

- Symptoms: Discussing the specific symptoms you're experiencing, their duration, and their severity.
- Family History: Reviewing any family history of autoimmune disorders, thyroid issues, or other related conditions.
- Medical History: Providing information about your health history, including previous diagnoses and treatments, medications, and other medical conditions.
- Physical Examination: The provider may perform a physical examination, including palpating the neck to assess the size and texture of the thyroid gland.

Based on the information gathered, the provider may recommend further testing to confirm a diagnosis.

DIAGNOSTIC TESTS

A range of diagnostic tests may be performed to assess thyroid function and identify autoimmune activity in the thyroid:

- Thyroid-Stimulating Hormone (TSH): TSH is produced by the pituitary gland and stimulates the thyroid gland to produce thyroid hormones. Elevated TSH levels can indicate hypothyroidism, a sign of Hashimoto's.

- Free T4 and T3: These tests measure the levels of the active thyroid hormones, thyroxine (T4) and triiodothyronine (T3). Low levels suggest an underactive thyroid.

- Thyroid Peroxidase Antibodies (TPOAb): This test measures antibodies against thyroid peroxidase, an enzyme involved in hormone production. Elevated levels indicate an autoimmune attack on the thyroid.

- Thyroglobulin Antibodies (TgAb): This test measures antibodies against thyroglobulin, a protein involved in thyroid hormone production. High levels suggest autoimmune activity against the thyroid.

- Ultrasound: An ultrasound of the thyroid gland can assess its size, structure, and detect any nodules or abnormalities. It can also help evaluate the presence of inflammation or an enlarged thyroid (goiter).

Additional tests may be performed depending on the individual's symptoms and medical history.

CHALLENGES IN DIAGNOSIS

Diagnosing Hashimoto's can present several challenges:

- Nonspecific Symptoms: Many of the symptoms of Hashimoto's, such as fatigue and mood changes, are nonspecific and can overlap with other conditions.
- Fluctuating Symptoms: Symptoms may fluctuate over time, making it difficult to recognize a consistent pattern indicative of Hashimoto's.
- Normal Thyroid Levels: In the early stages of Hashimoto's, TSH and thyroid hormone levels may be within the normal range, potentially delaying diagnosis.
- Misdiagnosis: Due to the overlap with other conditions, individuals with Hashimoto's may be misdiagnosed with depression, chronic fatigue syndrome, or other disorders before the thyroid condition is identified.

IMPORTANCE OF EARLY DIAGNOSIS

Early diagnosis of Hashimoto's is essential for effective management and prevention of further thyroid damage. Identifying the condition in its early stages allows for timely treatment and monitoring, reducing the risk of complications.

- Preventing Complications: Left untreated, Hashimoto's can lead to severe hypothyroidism, which may cause heart problems, infertility, and other health issues.

- Improving Quality of Life: Early intervention can help alleviate symptoms and improve overall well-being and quality of life.

- Guiding Treatment: Accurate diagnosis guides treatment decisions, including the appropriate medication and lifestyle adjustments.

WORKING WITH HEALTHCARE PROVIDERS

Collaborating closely with healthcare providers is key to obtaining an accurate diagnosis and developing an effective treatment plan. Open communication and asking questions can help ensure that you receive the best possible care:

- Advocate for Yourself: If you suspect you have Hashimoto's, discuss your concerns with your healthcare provider and request the necessary tests.

- Seek a Specialist: Consider consulting an endocrinologist, who specializes in thyroid disorders, for a more in-depth evaluation and treatment options.

- Stay Informed: Educate yourself about the condition and potential treatment options to actively participate in your care.

Conclusion

Diagnosing Hashimoto's thyroiditis involves a thorough assessment of symptoms, medical history, and diagnostic tests. While the process can be challenging, early diagnosis is crucial for effective management and improved quality of life. Collaborating closely with healthcare providers and staying informed about the condition can empower you to take charge of your health journey.

This chapter covers the process of diagnosing Hashimoto's thyroiditis, including initial consultations, diagnostic tests, and the importance of early diagnosis. The following chapters will delve into treatment options, lifestyle adjustments, and coping strategies to navigate your journey with Hashimoto's.

CHAPTER 4: TREATMENT AND MANAGEMENT OPTIONS

OVERVIEW OF TREATMENT

Treatment for Hashimoto's thyroiditis typically focuses on hormone replacement therapy to restore thyroid hormone levels to a healthy range. Managing Hashimoto's also involves addressing symptoms and potential complications while adopting lifestyle changes to support overall health and well-being.

HORMONE REPLACEMENT THERAPY

The primary treatment for Hashimoto's is hormone replacement therapy, which involves taking medication to replace the hormones the thyroid gland is unable to produce in sufficient amounts.

- Levothyroxine (T4): Levothyroxine is a synthetic form of thyroxine (T4), the main hormone produced by the thyroid gland. It is the most common medication prescribed for Hashimoto's. Levothyroxine is usually taken orally in tablet form, and the dosage is tailored to the individual's needs based on blood tests and symptoms.

- Liothyronine (T3): In some cases, a synthetic form of triiodothyronine (T3), known as liothyronine, may be prescribed. This is less common and is usually considered when levothyroxine alone does not adequately control symptoms.

DOSAGE AND MONITORING

The goal of hormone replacement therapy is to maintain thyroid hormone levels within a normal range. Initial dosing is based on age, weight, and severity of hypothyroidism. Regular monitoring of thyroid hormone levels is necessary to adjust the dosage as needed. Blood tests, including TSH, free T4, and free T3, are typically conducted every 6-12 months to assess hormone levels and ensure the medication is working effectively.

SIDE EFFECTS AND INTERACTIONS

Levothyroxine is generally well-tolerated, but some individuals may experience side effects such as heart palpitations, anxiety, or insomnia if the dosage is too high. It's important to follow the healthcare provider's instructions and report any unusual symptoms.

Levothyroxine may interact with other medications, supplements, and certain foods, such as calcium or iron supplements, which can affect its absorption. Always inform your healthcare provider of any other medications or supplements you are taking.

ADDITIONAL MEDICATIONS AND TREATMENTS

In addition to hormone replacement therapy, other medications may be considered depending on the individual's symptoms and health needs:

- Beta-Blockers: These medications may be prescribed to manage symptoms such as rapid heart rate and tremors, particularly in the early stages of treatment.

- Anti-Inflammatories: Nonsteroidal anti-inflammatory drugs (NSAIDs) may help manage inflammation and pain associated with thyroiditis.

- Selenium Supplements: Selenium is an essential mineral for thyroid function, and supplementation may help reduce thyroid inflammation in some individuals.

LIFESTYLE CHANGES

Adopting healthy lifestyle habits can complement medical treatment and support overall health:

- Nutrition: A balanced diet rich in essential nutrients, including iodine, selenium, zinc, and iron, can support thyroid function. Avoiding foods that interfere with thyroid hormone absorption, such as soy and high-fiber foods, may be beneficial.

- Exercise: Regular physical activity can help manage weight, boost energy levels, and improve mood. Exercise should be tailored to the individual's abilities and comfort level.

- Stress Management: Chronic stress can exacerbate symptoms. Techniques such as mindfulness, meditation, or yoga can help manage stress and support emotional well-being.

- Adequate Sleep: Prioritizing quality sleep is important for overall health and helps manage fatigue and mood changes.

ALTERNATIVE AND COMPLEMENTARY THERAPIES

While hormone replacement therapy is the primary treatment for Hashimoto's, some individuals may explore alternative and complementary therapies:

- Acupuncture: Acupuncture may help manage stress, improve sleep, and alleviate certain symptoms.

- Herbal Supplements: Certain herbal supplements, such as ashwagandha, may support thyroid health, but their efficacy varies, and they should be used with caution and under medical supervision.

- Chiropractic Care: Chiropractic adjustments may help relieve neck pain and tension, which can be beneficial for individuals with goiter.

It's essential to discuss any alternative or complementary therapies with your healthcare provider to ensure they are safe and compatible with your existing treatment plan.

SUPPORTIVE CARE AND COPING STRATEGIES

Living with Hashimoto's can present emotional and psychological challenges. Seeking support and finding coping strategies can improve quality of life:

- Support Groups: Joining support groups, either in person or online, can provide a sense of community and understanding.
- Counseling: Speaking with a therapist or counselor can help manage emotional challenges, anxiety, or depression.
- Education: Educating yourself about Hashimoto's can empower you to take an active role in your health and treatment decisions.

Conclusion

Treatment and management of Hashimoto's involve hormone replacement therapy, lifestyle changes, and supportive care. Collaborating closely with healthcare providers and staying informed about the condition can help you navigate your journey with Hashimoto's and improve your quality of life.

This chapter covers the treatment and management options for Hashimoto's thyroiditis, including hormone replacement therapy, lifestyle changes, and complementary therapies. Subsequent chapters will delve into personal experiences and strategies for coping with the challenges of living with Hashimoto's.

CHAPTER 5: NAVIGATING LIFE WITH HASHIMOTO'S

THE EMOTIONAL IMPACT OF HASHIMOTO'S

Living with Hashimoto's thyroiditis can have a significant emotional impact on individuals due to the chronic nature of the condition and the array of symptoms it presents. Here are some common emotional challenges faced by those with Hashimoto's:

- Anxiety and Depression: Hormonal imbalances and the chronic nature of the condition can contribute to anxiety and depression. These mood disorders can affect daily life and relationships.

- Frustration and Fatigue: The persistent fatigue and fluctuations in symptoms can lead to frustration and a sense of helplessness.

- Body Image Issues: Weight changes, hair loss, and skin changes can impact body image and self-esteem.

- Isolation: Individuals may feel isolated due to difficulty explaining their condition to others or because symptoms limit social interactions.

BUILDING A SUPPORT SYSTEM

A strong support system can make a significant difference in managing the emotional and physical challenges of Hashimoto's:

- Family and Friends: Educate your loved ones about your condition so they can understand your challenges and offer support.
- Support Groups: Joining a support group, either in person or online, can provide a sense of community and a safe space to share experiences and advice.
- Counseling: Seeking professional counseling can help manage emotional challenges and provide coping strategies for living with Hashimoto's.

COPING STRATEGIES

Developing effective coping strategies can help individuals navigate the challenges of Hashimoto's:

- Mindfulness and Meditation: Practices such as meditation and mindfulness can help manage stress and improve emotional well-being.
- Journaling: Writing about your experiences can help process emotions and track symptoms, which can be useful in discussions with healthcare providers.
- Creative Outlets: Engaging in creative activities such as art, music, or writing can provide an outlet for expression and help alleviate stress.
- Physical Activity: Regular exercise can boost mood, improve energy levels, and support overall health. Choose activities that you enjoy and that are within your comfort level.

MANAGING WORK AND CAREER

Hashimoto's can affect work and career due to symptoms such as fatigue, cognitive impairment, and mood changes. Here are some strategies to manage work life:

- Communicate with Your Employer: Discuss your condition with your employer to explore possible accommodations, such as flexible hours or remote work.

- Manage Energy Levels: Prioritize tasks based on your energy levels, and take breaks as needed to rest and recharge.

- Organize and Plan: Use organizational tools and planners to manage tasks and deadlines, allowing for adjustments as needed based on your symptoms.

NAVIGATING RELATIONSHIPS

Hashimoto's can impact personal relationships due to mood swings, fatigue, and changes in physical appearance. Here's how to navigate these challenges:

- Communicate Openly: Share your experiences and challenges with your partner, family, and friends. Open communication can foster understanding and empathy.

- Set Boundaries: Establish boundaries around your energy and emotional capacity, and communicate them to your loved ones.

- Seek Support: Counseling and support groups can provide guidance on navigating relationship challenges.

PARENTHOOD AND FAMILY PLANNING

For individuals with Hashimoto's who are considering parenthood, there are important factors to consider:

- Fertility: Thyroid hormone imbalances can affect fertility. Work closely with a healthcare provider to optimize thyroid levels before and during pregnancy.

- Pregnancy: Hashimoto's can impact pregnancy, so it's important to monitor thyroid levels throughout pregnancy to ensure the health of both mother and baby.

- Postpartum Thyroiditis: Some individuals may experience postpartum thyroiditis, a temporary thyroid disorder following childbirth. Monitor symptoms and seek medical advice if needed.

Conclusion

Navigating life with Hashimoto's thyroiditis involves managing the emotional impact, building a support system, and developing coping strategies. Open communication with loved ones, healthcare providers, and employers can help individuals thrive while living with Hashimoto's. Understanding the condition and finding effective ways to manage symptoms can lead to an improved quality of life.

This chapter explores navigating life with Hashimoto's, including the emotional impact, support systems, coping strategies, work and relationship challenges, and considerations for parenthood. Subsequent chapters will provide additional insights into specific aspects of living with Hashimoto's and practical advice for thriving with the condition.

CHAPTER 6: NUTRITION AND DIET FOR HASHIMOTO'S

THE ROLE OF NUTRITION IN MANAGING HASHIMOTO'S

Proper nutrition plays a crucial role in managing Hashimoto's thyroiditis and supporting overall health. A well-balanced diet can help manage symptoms, support thyroid function, and improve quality of life. While there is no one-size-fits-all diet for Hashimoto's, certain dietary approaches and nutrient considerations can be beneficial.

KEY NUTRIENTS FOR THYROID HEALTH

Several nutrients are essential for thyroid function and overall health:

- Iodine: Iodine is a key component of thyroid hormones. However, excessive iodine intake can exacerbate Hashimoto's, so it's important to maintain a balanced intake. Good sources include iodized salt, dairy products, and seafood.

- Selenium: Selenium is essential for thyroid hormone synthesis and helps regulate the immune system. Good sources include Brazil nuts, eggs, fish, and whole grains.

- Zinc: Zinc supports the immune system and thyroid function. Good sources include meat, shellfish, legumes, and nuts.

- Iron: Iron is crucial for thyroid hormone production and metabolism. Good sources include red meat, poultry, fish, and fortified cereals.

FOODS TO INCLUDE

Incorporating certain foods into your diet can support thyroid health and overall well-being:

- Fruits and Vegetables: A variety of colorful fruits and vegetables provide essential vitamins, minerals, and antioxidants that support the immune system and overall health.

- Whole Grains: Whole grains such as quinoa, brown rice, and oats provide fiber and essential nutrients.

- Lean Proteins: Sources of lean protein such as poultry, fish, and legumes can help maintain energy levels and support muscle health.

- Healthy Fats: Incorporate sources of healthy fats such as avocados, nuts, seeds, and olive oil for their anti-inflammatory and nutrient-rich properties.

- Probiotic-Rich Foods: Foods like yogurt, kefir, and sauerkraut can support gut health and immune function.

FOODS TO LIMIT OR AVOID

Certain foods may interfere with thyroid function or exacerbate symptoms and should be limited or avoided:

- Goitrogens: Goitrogens are compounds found in cruciferous vegetables like broccoli, cabbage, and Brussels sprouts. Cooking these vegetables can reduce their goitrogenic effects.

- Soy: Soy and soy-based products may interfere with thyroid hormone absorption, so it's best to consume them in moderation.

- Gluten: Some individuals with Hashimoto's may have a sensitivity to gluten, which can exacerbate autoimmune activity. Consider a gluten-free diet if you suspect gluten sensitivity.

- Sugar and Processed Foods: High sugar intake and processed foods can contribute to inflammation and negatively impact overall health.

- Excessive Caffeine: Too much caffeine can interfere with sleep and exacerbate anxiety or palpitations, so moderate your intake.

DIETARY APPROACHES

Different dietary approaches can be helpful for managing Hashimoto's, but it's important to find the one that works best for you:

- Autoimmune Protocol (AIP): The AIP diet focuses on eliminating foods that may trigger inflammation or autoimmune reactions and reintroducing them gradually.

- Gluten-Free Diet: Eliminating gluten from your diet may help reduce autoimmune activity and improve symptoms.

- Paleo Diet: The paleo diet emphasizes whole foods and avoids grains, dairy, and processed foods, which may support thyroid health.

MEAL PLANNING AND PREPARATION

Planning and preparing meals can help you maintain a balanced diet and avoid foods that may negatively impact your health:

- Plan Ahead: Plan your meals in advance to ensure you're including a variety of nutrient-rich foods and avoiding trigger foods.
- Batch Cooking: Preparing meals in batches can save time and ensure you have healthy options available throughout the week.
- Listen to Your Body: Pay attention to how different foods make you feel and adjust your diet accordingly.

SUPPLEMENTS AND CONSIDERATIONS

In some cases, supplements may be necessary to support thyroid health and overall well-being:

- Multivitamins: A high-quality multivitamin can provide essential nutrients that may be lacking in your diet.
- Vitamin D: Many individuals with Hashimoto's have low vitamin D levels, which can affect immune function. Supplementation may be necessary if you are deficient.
- Omega-3 Fatty Acids: Omega-3 supplements can support anti-inflammatory processes and overall health.

Always consult your healthcare provider before starting any new supplements to ensure they are safe and appropriate for your specific needs.

Conclusion

Nutrition and diet play a crucial role in managing Hashimoto's thyroiditis and supporting overall health. By focusing on a balanced diet rich in key nutrients, avoiding trigger foods, and considering specific dietary approaches, you can support thyroid function and improve your quality of life. Collaborate with a healthcare provider or registered dietitian to create a personalized nutrition plan that works best for you.

This chapter covers the role of nutrition and diet in managing Hashimoto's thyroiditis, including key nutrients, foods to include and avoid, dietary approaches, and meal planning tips. Subsequent chapters will delve into additional strategies for thriving with Hashimoto's and practical advice for managing the condition.

CHAPTER 7: EXERCISE AND PHYSICAL ACTIVITY WITH HASHIMOTO'S

THE IMPORTANCE OF PHYSICAL ACTIVITY

Exercise and physical activity are essential components of a healthy lifestyle for individuals with Hashimoto's thyroiditis. Regular exercise can help manage symptoms, support overall health, and improve quality of life. However, it's important to approach physical activity with consideration for individual energy levels and limitations.

BENEFITS OF EXERCISE

Engaging in regular physical activity can offer numerous benefits for individuals with Hashimoto's:

- Improved Energy Levels: Exercise can boost energy and combat fatigue by promoting circulation and enhancing mitochondrial function.

- Weight Management: Maintaining a healthy weight is important for thyroid health. Exercise can support weight loss or maintenance goals.

- Mood Enhancement: Physical activity can increase the production of endorphins and serotonin, improving mood and reducing symptoms of anxiety and depression.

- Heart Health: Cardiovascular exercise can improve heart health, which is important for individuals with thyroid issues that may affect heart rate and rhythm.

- Bone Health: Weight-bearing exercise supports bone density, helping prevent osteoporosis, which is more common in individuals with Hashimoto's.

TYPES OF EXERCISE

Various types of exercise can benefit individuals with Hashimoto's, and the choice of activities should be based on personal preferences, fitness level, and energy levels:

- Cardiovascular Exercise: Activities like walking, swimming, cycling, and dancing can improve heart health and endurance.
- Strength Training: Resistance exercises, such as weightlifting or bodyweight exercises, can help maintain muscle mass and improve metabolism.
- Flexibility and Mobility: Stretching, yoga, and Pilates can improve flexibility and mobility, reducing stiffness and muscle tension.
- Mind-Body Practices: Practices like yoga and tai chi can promote relaxation, reduce stress, and improve overall well-being.

CREATING AN EXERCISE PLAN

Developing a personalized exercise plan can help you stay active while considering your unique needs and limitations:

- Start Slowly: If you're new to exercise or have been inactive for a while, start with low-intensity activities and gradually increase intensity and duration.

- Listen to Your Body: Pay attention to your body's signals and adjust your exercise plan based on how you feel. Rest when needed and avoid overexertion.

- Set Realistic Goals: Establish achievable exercise goals based on your fitness level and health needs. Celebrate your progress and achievements.

- Consistency is Key: Aim for regular physical activity, even if it's just a short walk each day. Consistency can lead to long-term health benefits.

MANAGING EXERCISE-INDUCED FATIGUE

Fatigue can be a significant challenge for individuals with Hashimoto's, particularly after exercise. Here are some strategies to manage exercise-induced fatigue:

- Pace Yourself: Choose activities and durations that match your energy levels, and take breaks when needed.
- Stay Hydrated: Proper hydration can help maintain energy levels and prevent dehydration, which can exacerbate fatigue.
- Fuel Your Body: Eating a balanced diet with adequate protein and healthy carbohydrates can provide sustained energy for physical activity.
- Prioritize Rest and Recovery: Allow your body time to rest and recover between workouts to prevent burnout and overexertion.

SAFETY CONSIDERATIONS

Safety should always be a priority when engaging in physical activity:

- Consult Your Healthcare Provider: Before starting a new exercise program, consult your healthcare provider to ensure it's safe and appropriate for your specific health needs.

- Warm Up and Cool Down: Always include a proper warm-up and cool-down in your exercise routine to prepare your body and prevent injury.

- Listen to Your Body: Pay attention to any unusual symptoms during exercise, such as chest pain or shortness of breath, and seek medical advice if necessary.

- Choose Suitable Activities: Opt for exercises that are low-impact and gentle on the joints to minimize the risk of injury.

Conclusion

Exercise and physical activity are essential components of managing Hashimoto's thyroiditis and supporting overall health. By engaging in a variety of activities and listening to your body's needs, you can reap the benefits of exercise while minimizing the risks of fatigue and injury. Collaborate with your healthcare provider to create an exercise plan that works best for you and supports your journey to thriving with Hashimoto's.

This chapter explores the importance of exercise and physical activity for individuals with Hashimoto's thyroiditis, including the benefits, types of exercise, creating an exercise plan, managing fatigue, and safety considerations. Subsequent chapters will delve into additional strategies for thriving with Hashimoto's and practical advice for managing the condition.

CHAPTER 8: STRESS MANAGEMENT AND MENTAL HEALTH

THE CONNECTION BETWEEN STRESS AND HASHIMOTO'S

Stress can have a significant impact on individuals with Hashimoto's thyroiditis. Chronic stress may exacerbate symptoms and lead to hormone imbalances by disrupting the delicate relationship between the endocrine and immune systems. Managing stress effectively is crucial for overall health and quality of life for those with Hashimoto's.

UNDERSTANDING THE EFFECTS OF STRESS

Prolonged stress can affect the body in various ways:

- Hormonal Imbalance: Chronic stress can disrupt the hypothalamic-pituitary-adrenal (HPA) axis, affecting cortisol and other hormone levels.
- Immune System Dysregulation: Stress can lead to immune system dysregulation, potentially exacerbating autoimmune activity and inflammation.
- Mood Disorders: Stress can contribute to anxiety and depression, which are common comorbidities in Hashimoto's patients.
- Physical Symptoms: Stress can trigger or worsen physical symptoms such as fatigue, insomnia, muscle tension, and headaches.

EFFECTIVE STRESS MANAGEMENT TECHNIQUES

Adopting stress management techniques can help reduce the impact of stress on your health and improve your quality of life:

- Mindfulness and Meditation: Practicing mindfulness and meditation can help calm the mind, reduce stress, and improve emotional well-being.

- Deep Breathing: Deep breathing exercises, such as diaphragmatic breathing, can activate the parasympathetic nervous system, promoting relaxation and reducing stress.

- Progressive Muscle Relaxation: This technique involves tensing and relaxing different muscle groups to release physical tension and induce relaxation.

- Journaling: Writing about your experiences and emotions can help process stress and provide clarity on challenges and achievements.

- Time Management: Prioritizing tasks, setting boundaries, and organizing your schedule can help reduce stress and improve productivity.

EMOTIONAL WELL-BEING AND SELF-CARE

Caring for your emotional well-being is just as important as managing physical symptoms:

- Seek Counseling: Talking to a therapist or counselor can provide support and coping strategies for managing stress and emotional challenges.
- Practice Gratitude: Focusing on the positives in your life and practicing gratitude can improve mood and perspective.
- Engage in Activities You Enjoy: Pursuing hobbies and interests can provide a sense of fulfillment and relaxation.
- Connect with Loved Ones: Spending time with supportive family and friends can improve emotional well-being and reduce feelings of isolation.

SLEEP AND STRESS MANAGEMENT

Quality sleep is essential for managing stress and maintaining overall health:

- Establish a Bedtime Routine: Creating a consistent bedtime routine can help signal to your body that it's time to wind down.

- Limit Stimulants: Avoid caffeine and electronic devices close to bedtime to improve sleep quality.

- Create a Comfortable Sleep Environment: Ensure your bedroom is conducive to sleep, with a comfortable mattress, pillows, and a cool, dark, and quiet environment.

- Practice Relaxation Techniques: Relaxation exercises such as meditation, deep breathing, or gentle yoga can help calm the mind before sleep.

SEEKING SUPPORT

Building a support network can provide emotional and practical support for managing stress:

- Support Groups: Joining support groups, either in person or online, can offer a sense of community and shared experiences.

- Family and Friends: Communicate openly with your loved ones about your challenges and needs so they can provide support and understanding.

- Healthcare Provider: Consult your healthcare provider for advice on managing stress and mental health, and seek appropriate referrals if needed.

Conclusion

Effective stress management is essential for individuals with Hashimoto's thyroiditis to maintain overall health and improve quality of life. By adopting stress-reduction techniques, prioritizing emotional well-being, and seeking support, you can navigate the challenges of Hashimoto's more effectively and thrive with the condition.

This chapter explores the connection between stress and Hashimoto's, effective stress management techniques, and the importance of emotional well-being and self-care. Subsequent chapters will provide additional strategies and advice for thriving with Hashimoto's and managing the condition effectively.

CHAPTER 9: MEDICATION AND TREATMENT OPTIONS

UNDERSTANDING MEDICATION AND TREATMENT

Managing Hashimoto's thyroiditis often involves a combination of medication, lifestyle changes, and ongoing monitoring to ensure optimal thyroid function and overall health. This chapter will discuss the various medication and treatment options available for Hashimoto's and how to work with your healthcare provider to find the best approach for your needs.

THYROID HORMONE REPLACEMENT THERAPY

Thyroid hormone replacement therapy is a common treatment for individuals with Hashimoto's who experience hypothyroidism. The goal is to replace the deficient thyroid hormones and restore hormone levels to a normal range. There are several types of thyroid hormone replacement medications:

- Levothyroxine (T4): Levothyroxine is a synthetic form of thyroxine (T4), the main hormone produced by the thyroid gland. It's the most commonly prescribed thyroid hormone replacement medication.

- Liothyronine (T3): Liothyronine is a synthetic form of triiodothyronine (T3), a more active thyroid hormone. It may be used in combination with levothyroxine for individuals who do not respond well to T4-only therapy.

- Natural Desiccated Thyroid (NDT): NDT is derived from animal thyroid glands and contains both T4 and T3. Some individuals prefer NDT for its natural composition.

FINDING THE RIGHT DOSAGE

Finding the right dosage of thyroid hormone replacement medication is crucial for managing Hashimoto's and avoiding symptoms of under- or over-treatment:

- Regular Monitoring: Your healthcare provider will monitor your thyroid hormone levels regularly through blood tests to ensure your medication dosage is appropriate.

- Symptom Assessment: In addition to lab results, your healthcare provider will assess your symptoms and overall well-being to adjust your medication dosage if needed.

- Patience and Adjustments: It may take time to find the right dosage and make adjustments as needed. Patience and open communication with your healthcare provider are key.

ADDITIONAL MEDICATIONS AND SUPPLEMENTS

In addition to thyroid hormone replacement therapy, other medications and supplements may be used to manage symptoms and support overall health:

- Anti-Inflammatory Medications: Nonsteroidal anti-inflammatory drugs (NSAIDs) may help manage pain and inflammation associated with Hashimoto's.
- Corticosteroids: In severe cases of inflammation, corticosteroids may be prescribed to reduce immune system activity and inflammation.
- Vitamin D and Iron Supplements: Vitamin D and iron deficiencies are common in individuals with Hashimoto's. Supplements may be recommended to correct these deficiencies.
- Selenium Supplements: Selenium supplementation may support thyroid function and reduce antibody levels in some individuals.

COMPLEMENTARY AND ALTERNATIVE TREATMENTS

Complementary and alternative treatments may be used alongside conventional treatments to support overall well-being:

- Acupuncture: Acupuncture may help alleviate symptoms such as fatigue, pain, and stress.

- Herbal Supplements: Some individuals may benefit from herbal supplements such as ashwagandha, which may support thyroid function and reduce stress. Always consult your healthcare provider before starting any new supplements.

- Naturopathy and Functional Medicine: These approaches may focus on personalized treatment plans that incorporate dietary changes, supplements, and lifestyle modifications.

WORKING WITH YOUR HEALTHCARE PROVIDER

Collaboration with your healthcare provider is essential for managing Hashimoto's and finding the most effective treatment plan:

- Communicate Openly: Share your symptoms, concerns, and treatment preferences with your healthcare provider.

- Ask Questions: Don't hesitate to ask questions about your treatment options, potential side effects, and expected outcomes.

- Stay Informed: Educate yourself about Hashimoto's and available treatment options to make informed decisions about your care.

- Monitor Your Health: Keep track of your symptoms and medication usage to help your healthcare provider make informed adjustments to your treatment plan.

Conclusion

Medication and treatment options are essential components of managing Hashimoto's thyroiditis and maintaining overall health. By working closely with your healthcare provider and exploring different treatment approaches, you can find the best plan for your needs and improve your quality of life.

This chapter explores medication and treatment options for managing Hashimoto's thyroiditis, including thyroid hormone replacement therapy, additional medications and supplements, complementary and alternative treatments, and the importance of working with your healthcare provider. Subsequent chapters will delve into other strategies and advice for thriving with Hashimoto's and managing the condition effectively.

CHAPTER 10: LIFESTYLE ADJUSTMENTS FOR LIVING WITH HASHIMOTO'S

Introduction

Living with Hashimoto's thyroiditis requires making certain lifestyle adjustments to manage symptoms, support thyroid function, and improve overall quality of life. This chapter will discuss practical lifestyle changes and strategies that can help individuals thrive while managing Hashimoto's.

BALANCING WORK AND REST

Achieving a balance between work and rest is essential for individuals with Hashimoto's:

- Prioritize Rest: Fatigue is a common symptom of Hashimoto's. Prioritize rest and listen to your body when you need to take breaks.
- Manage Workload: Adjust your workload to match your energy levels, and avoid overcommitting to tasks that may cause burnout.
- Set Boundaries: Establish clear boundaries at work and home to prevent overexertion and allow time for relaxation and recovery.

STAYING ACTIVE

Regular physical activity can improve overall health and well-being:

- Choose Enjoyable Activities: Find exercises you enjoy and can sustain long-term, such as walking, swimming, or yoga.
- Start Slowly: Begin with low-impact activities and gradually increase intensity and duration as your fitness level improves.
- Listen to Your Body: Pay attention to how your body responds to exercise and adjust your routine accordingly.

MANAGING WEIGHT AND NUTRITION

Maintaining a healthy weight and balanced diet is important for managing Hashimoto's:

- Monitor Your Diet: Pay attention to how different foods affect your symptoms and energy levels. Adjust your diet to include nutrient-dense foods and limit processed or inflammatory foods.
- Practice Portion Control: Be mindful of portion sizes and avoid overeating, which can contribute to weight gain and other health issues.
- Seek Professional Guidance: Consider consulting a registered dietitian or nutritionist for personalized dietary advice.

STRESS MANAGEMENT AND MENTAL HEALTH

Managing stress and prioritizing mental health is crucial for overall well-being:

- Adopt Stress-Reduction Techniques: Techniques such as mindfulness, meditation, deep breathing, and yoga can help manage stress and improve emotional well-being.
- Seek Support: Connect with supportive friends, family, or support groups to share experiences and gain emotional support.
- Practice Self-Care: Engage in activities that bring you joy and relaxation, such as reading, gardening, or listening to music.

SLEEP HYGIENE

Quality sleep is essential for managing symptoms and maintaining energy levels:

- Establish a Bedtime Routine: Create a consistent bedtime routine to signal to your body that it's time to wind down.

- Optimize Your Sleep Environment: Ensure your bedroom is conducive to sleep, with a comfortable mattress, pillows, and a cool, dark, and quiet environment.

- Limit Stimulants: Avoid caffeine and electronic devices close to bedtime to improve sleep quality.

SOCIAL AND EMOTIONAL SUPPORT

Building a strong support network can improve your overall quality of life:

- Communicate Openly: Share your experiences and challenges with loved ones to foster understanding and support.

- Join Support Groups: Connecting with others who have Hashimoto's can provide a sense of community and shared experiences.

- Seek Professional Help: If you experience persistent anxiety or depression, consider seeking the help of a therapist or counselor.

ENVIRONMENTAL CONSIDERATIONS

Certain environmental factors may impact thyroid health and overall well-being:

- Minimize Toxin Exposure: Limit exposure to environmental toxins such as pesticides, heavy metals, and pollutants, which may interfere with thyroid function.
- Choose Safe Personal Care Products: Opt for natural and non-toxic personal care products to reduce exposure to endocrine-disrupting chemicals.
- Filter Your Water: Use water filters to remove contaminants such as chlorine and fluoride, which may affect thyroid health.

MONITORING AND REGULAR CHECK-UPS

Ongoing monitoring and regular check-ups are essential for managing Hashimoto's:

- Track Your Symptoms: Keep a journal of your symptoms, medication use, and any changes in your condition to help your healthcare provider adjust your treatment plan.

- Attend Regular Check-Ups: Schedule regular appointments with your healthcare provider to monitor your thyroid function and overall health.

- Communicate Changes: Inform your healthcare provider of any changes in your symptoms or medication use to ensure optimal management.

Conclusion

Adopting lifestyle adjustments is key to managing Hashimoto's thyroiditis and thriving with the condition. By balancing work and rest, staying active, managing weight and nutrition, and prioritizing stress management and mental health, you can improve your quality of life and better manage your symptoms. Collaborate with your healthcare provider and seek support from loved ones and support groups to navigate the challenges of living with Hashimoto's effectively.

This chapter discusses various lifestyle adjustments individuals with Hashimoto's can make to manage symptoms and improve quality of life. Subsequent chapters will continue to provide additional strategies and advice for thriving with Hashimoto's and managing the condition effectively.

CHAPTER 11: BUILDING A SUPPORT NETWORK

Introduction

Building a strong support network is a vital part of managing Hashimoto's thyroiditis and thriving with the condition. A well-rounded network can provide emotional support, practical assistance, and valuable resources for navigating the challenges of living with an autoimmune thyroid disease.

THE IMPORTANCE OF A SUPPORT NETWORK

Having a support network can offer numerous benefits for individuals with Hashimoto's:

- Emotional Support: Connecting with others who understand your experiences can provide comfort, encouragement, and validation.

- Practical Assistance: Family and friends can offer help with daily tasks, appointments, and other responsibilities when you're experiencing symptoms such as fatigue.

- Sharing Information: A support network can share tips, resources, and advice on managing Hashimoto's, including dietary and lifestyle changes.

- Accountability: Being part of a support network can provide motivation and accountability for making positive changes and sticking to your treatment plan.

BUILDING YOUR SUPPORT NETWORK

Here are some strategies for building and nurturing a support network that meets your needs:

- Family and Friends: Share your experiences with loved ones so they can understand your condition and offer support. Educate them about Hashimoto's and how it affects your daily life.

- Support Groups: Joining support groups, either in person or online, can connect you with others who have similar experiences. Support groups offer a sense of community and understanding.

- Healthcare Professionals: Your healthcare team can provide guidance, treatment, and support. Communicate openly with them about your needs and any challenges you face.

- Online Communities: Online forums and social media groups can provide additional support and resources. Engage with these communities to share experiences and learn from others.

TYPES OF SUPPORT GROUPS

Support groups come in various forms and can be tailored to your preferences and needs:

- Local In-Person Groups: Many cities have local support groups for individuals with thyroid conditions. These groups provide face-to-face interaction and community support.

- Online Support Groups: Online groups and forums offer the convenience of connecting with others from the comfort of your home. They can be especially helpful for those in remote areas or with limited mobility.

- Condition-Specific Groups: Some support groups focus specifically on Hashimoto's or autoimmune thyroid conditions, providing targeted support and information.

- General Chronic Illness Groups: Broader support groups for individuals with chronic illnesses can also offer valuable insights and support.

NURTURING RELATIONSHIPS WITH LOVED ONES

Fostering strong relationships with family and friends is crucial for emotional and practical support:

- Communicate Openly: Share your feelings, experiences, and challenges with loved ones so they can understand your needs.

- Set Expectations: Help loved ones understand how Hashimoto's affects your energy levels and abilities, and set realistic expectations for your participation in activities.

- Show Appreciation: Express gratitude for the support you receive from family and friends. Acknowledge their efforts and let them know how much they mean to you.

SEEKING PROFESSIONAL SUPPORT

In addition to building a personal support network, seeking professional support can be beneficial:

• Therapists and Counselors: If you experience anxiety, depression, or other emotional challenges, consider seeing a therapist or counselor for professional guidance and support.

• Dietitians and Nutritionists: A registered dietitian or nutritionist can provide personalized dietary advice and support for managing Hashimoto's.

• Specialists: Endocrinologists or other specialists can offer expert medical advice and treatment for managing your condition.

Conclusion

Building a strong support network is essential for managing Hashimoto's thyroiditis and thriving with the condition. By nurturing relationships with family and friends, engaging with support groups, and seeking professional support when needed, you can create a supportive environment that empowers you to navigate the challenges of Hashimoto's more effectively and improve your overall quality of life.

This chapter discusses the importance of building a support network for individuals with Hashimoto's, including the benefits, types of support groups, and strategies for nurturing relationships. Subsequent chapters will continue to provide additional strategies and advice for thriving with Hashimoto's and managing the condition effectively.

CHAPTER 12: LONG-TERM MANAGEMENT AND MONITORING

Introduction

Long-term management and monitoring are essential aspects of living with Hashimoto's thyroiditis. Effective management involves regularly assessing thyroid function, maintaining consistent treatment, and making lifestyle adjustments to optimize overall health and well-being. This chapter will discuss strategies for long-term management and monitoring of Hashimoto's.

THE IMPORTANCE OF LONG-TERM MANAGEMENT

Ongoing management of Hashimoto's thyroiditis is important for several reasons:

- Stability of Thyroid Function: Regular monitoring helps ensure that thyroid hormone levels remain within a healthy range, reducing the risk of complications.
- Symptom Management: Long-term management helps control symptoms such as fatigue, weight changes, and mood swings.
- Prevention of Complications: Proper management can help prevent potential complications such as goiter, heart problems, and other autoimmune conditions.
- Quality of Life: Consistent management improves overall quality of life and supports the ability to engage in daily activities.

Regular Monitoring of Thyroid Function

Monitoring thyroid function is a key part of long-term management:

- Blood Tests: Regular blood tests, such as thyroid-stimulating hormone (TSH), free thyroxine (FT4), and free triiodothyronine (FT3), help assess thyroid hormone levels and guide treatment adjustments.

- Antibody Testing: Periodic testing for thyroid antibodies (anti-thyroid peroxidase and anti-thyroglobulin) can provide information about the autoimmune aspect of the condition.

- Symptom Assessment: Keep track of your symptoms and any changes over time. Share this information with your healthcare provider to aid in treatment adjustments.

ADJUSTING MEDICATION AND TREATMENT

Adjusting medication and treatment is sometimes necessary to maintain optimal thyroid function:

- Communicate with Your Healthcare Provider: Share any changes in symptoms or side effects with your healthcare provider to determine if medication adjustments are needed.

- Follow Up on Blood Test Results: Review blood test results with your healthcare provider to ensure your thyroid hormone levels are within the target range.

- Be Open to Treatment Changes: Your healthcare provider may recommend adjustments to your medication dosage or type over time. Stay open to changes as needed.

Lifestyle Modifications for Long-Term Management

Lifestyle modifications play a significant role in long-term management of Hashimoto's:

- Balanced Diet: Maintain a balanced diet rich in nutrients that support thyroid function, such as iodine, selenium, and zinc.

- Regular Exercise: Engage in regular physical activity that you enjoy and can sustain long-term. Adjust exercise intensity based on your energy levels and overall health.

- Stress Management: Practice stress-reduction techniques such as mindfulness, meditation, or yoga to support mental and emotional well-being.

- Sleep Hygiene: Prioritize quality sleep by establishing a consistent sleep schedule and creating a relaxing bedtime routine.

PREVENTING COMPLICATIONS

Preventing complications associated with Hashimoto's is a key aspect of long-term management:

- Monitor Other Health Conditions: Individuals with Hashimoto's are at an increased risk of other autoimmune conditions. Regular check-ups can help detect and manage any additional health issues.

- Manage Cardiovascular Health: Thyroid dysfunction can affect heart health. Monitor blood pressure, cholesterol levels, and heart rate regularly.

- Bone Health: Hypothyroidism can affect bone density. Ensure adequate intake of calcium and vitamin D and consider bone density tests as recommended.

BUILDING A SUPPORT NETWORK

Maintaining a strong support network can enhance long-term management:

- Stay Connected: Keep in touch with supportive family and friends who understand your condition and can provide emotional support.
- Engage with Support Groups: Participate in support groups, either in person or online, to share experiences and learn from others with Hashimoto's.
- Consult Healthcare Professionals: Regularly consult your healthcare provider for ongoing monitoring and treatment adjustments.

Conclusion

Long-term management and monitoring are essential for living well with Hashimoto's thyroiditis. By regularly assessing thyroid function, adjusting treatment as needed, and making lifestyle modifications, you can optimize your overall health and quality of life. Building a strong support network and maintaining open communication with your healthcare provider are key components of successful long-term management.

This chapter discusses long-term management and monitoring strategies for individuals with Hashimoto's, including regular monitoring of thyroid function, adjusting medication and treatment, lifestyle modifications, preventing complications, and building a support network. Subsequent chapters will continue to provide additional strategies and advice for thriving with Hashimoto's and managing the condition effectively.

CHAPTER 13: COPING WITH HASHIMOTO'S AND DAILY LIFE

Introduction

Living with Hashimoto's thyroiditis presents unique challenges that can impact daily life, from managing symptoms to balancing work and personal responsibilities. In this chapter, we will explore strategies for coping with Hashimoto's and maintaining a fulfilling daily life despite the condition.

NAVIGATING DAILY ACTIVITIES

Finding ways to manage daily activities while dealing with symptoms is key to maintaining a good quality of life:

- Prioritize and Plan: Identify your most important tasks and tackle them when your energy levels are highest. Plan your day around periods of productivity and rest.
- Delegate When Possible: Enlist the help of family, friends, or coworkers for tasks that may be challenging during flare-ups.
- Pace Yourself: Break tasks into smaller, manageable steps and take breaks as needed to avoid overexertion.

WORK-LIFE BALANCE

Maintaining a healthy work-life balance is crucial for managing Hashimoto's:

- Communicate with Your Employer: If needed, discuss accommodations or adjustments at work with your employer to help manage your condition.

- Set Boundaries: Establish clear boundaries between work and personal life to prevent burnout and maintain energy for other important activities.

- Use Flexible Work Arrangements: If available, explore flexible work options such as telecommuting or flexible hours to better accommodate your needs.

COPING WITH FATIGUE

Fatigue is a common symptom of Hashimoto's and can significantly impact daily life:

- Prioritize Rest: Ensure you get enough rest and sleep each night to manage fatigue and support overall health.
- Take Naps: Short naps during the day can help recharge your energy levels and improve focus.
- Listen to Your Body: Pay attention to your body's signals and adjust your activities to avoid pushing yourself too hard.

EMOTIONAL WELL-BEING

Coping with Hashimoto's can take a toll on emotional well-being. Prioritizing mental health is essential:

- Seek Support: Talk to loved ones or a therapist about your experiences and emotions. Sharing your feelings can provide relief and perspective.

- Practice Stress Management: Engage in stress-reduction techniques such as meditation, deep breathing exercises, or yoga to promote relaxation and emotional balance.

- Stay Connected: Maintain social connections with friends and family to combat feelings of isolation and provide emotional support.

MANAGING RELATIONSHIPS

Hashimoto's can affect relationships with others, so it's important to communicate openly:

- Educate Loved Ones: Help loved ones understand your condition and its impact on your daily life.
- Be Honest About Limitations: Share your limitations and challenges with those close to you to set realistic expectations.
- Express Gratitude: Show appreciation for the support you receive from loved ones to strengthen your relationships.

OVERCOMING BRAIN FOG

Hashimoto's can cause brain fog, affecting memory, concentration, and cognitive function:

- Stay Organized: Use calendars, lists, and reminders to keep track of important tasks and appointments.
- Take Breaks: Give your mind regular breaks to rest and recharge.
- Engage in Brain-Boosting Activities: Puzzles, reading, and other stimulating activities can help improve cognitive function.

DIET AND NUTRITION

A healthy diet can help manage symptoms and support overall health:

- Focus on Nutrient-Dense Foods: Choose whole, unprocessed foods rich in vitamins and minerals.
- Stay Hydrated: Drink plenty of water throughout the day to stay hydrated and support bodily functions.
- Consider Food Sensitivities: Some individuals with Hashimoto's may have sensitivities to certain foods, such as gluten or dairy. Pay attention to your body's response to different foods and adjust your diet accordingly.

Conclusion

Coping with Hashimoto's and daily life requires flexibility, patience, and self-awareness. By navigating daily activities strategically, maintaining a healthy work-life balance, prioritizing emotional well-being, and adjusting your diet, you can manage symptoms and maintain a fulfilling daily life. Continuously assess your needs and make adjustments as necessary to thrive while living with Hashimoto's.

This chapter explores strategies for coping with Hashimoto's and daily life, including navigating daily activities, maintaining work-life balance, managing fatigue, prioritizing emotional well-being, overcoming brain fog, and adjusting diet and nutrition. Subsequent chapters will continue to provide additional strategies and advice for thriving with Hashimoto's and managing the condition effectively.

CHAPTER 14: EXPLORING COMPLEMENTARY AND ALTERNATIVE THERAPIES

Introduction

In addition to conventional medical treatments, complementary and alternative therapies can play a role in managing Hashimoto's thyroiditis and its symptoms. While these therapies should not replace prescribed treatments, they can enhance overall well-being and support the management of Hashimoto's. This chapter will discuss various complementary and alternative therapies that individuals with Hashimoto's may find beneficial.

UNDERSTANDING COMPLEMENTARY AND ALTERNATIVE THERAPIES

Complementary and alternative therapies encompass a wide range of practices and treatments:

- Complementary Therapies: These are non-mainstream therapies used alongside conventional medical treatments to support overall health and symptom management.

- Alternative Therapies: These are non-mainstream therapies used in place of conventional medical treatments.

It's important to consult with your healthcare provider before starting any complementary or alternative therapy to ensure its safety and effectiveness in your specific case.

ACUPUNCTURE

Acupuncture is a traditional Chinese medicine practice that involves inserting fine needles into specific points on the body:

- Benefits: Acupuncture may help alleviate symptoms such as fatigue, muscle pain, and anxiety. It is also known to promote relaxation and improve energy flow.

- Safety: When performed by a qualified practitioner, acupuncture is generally considered safe. Always ensure the practitioner is certified and follows proper hygiene practices.

HERBAL MEDICINE

Herbal medicine uses plants and plant extracts to support health and manage symptoms:

- Benefits: Some herbs may support thyroid function, reduce inflammation, or alleviate symptoms. For example, ashwagandha and guggul are known to have potential benefits for thyroid health.//- Caution: Herbal remedies can interact with medications or cause side effects. Consult with a healthcare provider or a qualified herbalist before using herbal supplements.

DIETARY SUPPLEMENTS

Dietary supplements, such as vitamins and minerals, can play a role in supporting thyroid health:

- Key Nutrients: Iodine, selenium, zinc, and vitamin D are important for thyroid function and overall health.
- Considerations: Speak with your healthcare provider before taking supplements to ensure appropriate dosages and avoid potential interactions with medications.

MIND-BODY PRACTICES

Mind-body practices such as yoga, meditation, and tai chi can help manage stress and improve overall well-being:

- Benefits: These practices promote relaxation, reduce stress, and improve mood. They can also help manage symptoms such as fatigue and anxiety.
- Customization: Mind-body practices can be tailored to individual preferences and abilities. Choose the techniques that resonate most with you.

MASSAGE THERAPY

Massage therapy involves manipulating the body's soft tissues to promote relaxation and alleviate tension:

- Benefits: Massage therapy may help reduce muscle tension, relieve stress, and improve circulation.
- Types of Massage: Different types of massage, such as Swedish, deep tissue, and lymphatic drainage, offer various benefits. Discuss your needs with a qualified massage therapist.

CHIROPRACTIC CARE

Chiropractic care focuses on the alignment of the spine and nervous system:

- Benefits: Chiropractic adjustments may help improve overall well-being, alleviate pain, and support nervous system function.
- Safety: Chiropractic care should be performed by a licensed practitioner. Discuss any concerns or limitations with your chiropractor.

AROMATHERAPY

Aromatherapy uses essential oils to promote relaxation and well-being:

- Benefits: Inhaling essential oils or using them topically may help manage symptoms such as anxiety and stress.
- Safety: Use essential oils with caution, as some oils may cause skin irritation or interact with medications. Dilute essential oils properly and consult with a healthcare provider if needed.

Conclusion

Exploring complementary and alternative therapies can enhance the overall management of Hashimoto's thyroiditis and improve quality of life. Always consult with your healthcare provider before starting any new therapy to ensure its safety and compatibility with your treatment plan. By incorporating these therapies thoughtfully, you can support your health and well-being while living with Hashimoto's.

This chapter discusses various complementary and alternative therapies that individuals with Hashimoto's may find beneficial, including acupuncture, herbal medicine, dietary supplements, mind-body practices, massage therapy, chiropractic care, and aromatherapy. Subsequent chapters will continue to provide additional strategies and advice for thriving with Hashimoto's and managing the condition effectively.

CHAPTER 15: COPING WITH SETBACKS AND FLARE-UPS

Introduction

Living with Hashimoto's thyroiditis can involve setbacks and flare-ups, where symptoms become more pronounced or new challenges arise. While setbacks can be frustrating, learning how to manage them effectively can help you regain control and minimize their impact on your life. In this chapter, we will discuss strategies for coping with setbacks and flare-ups, as well as how to maintain resilience during challenging times.

UNDERSTANDING SETBACKS AND FLARE-UPS

Setbacks and flare-ups can be caused by various factors, including:

•	Medication Changes: Adjustments in medication dosages or types can sometimes cause temporary disruptions in thyroid function.

•	Stress: Emotional, physical, or mental stress can exacerbate symptoms or trigger flare-ups.

•	Diet and Lifestyle: Changes in diet or lifestyle, such as poor sleep habits, can impact thyroid function.

•	Infections and Illnesses: Other illnesses or infections can worsen Hashimoto's symptoms.

COPING STRATEGIES FOR SETBACKS AND FLARE-UPS

Effective strategies can help you navigate setbacks and flare-ups more smoothly:

- **Stay Calm:** Try to remain calm and composed during a setback. Panicking can worsen stress and make symptoms more challenging to manage.

- **Identify Triggers:** Keep a symptom journal to track patterns and potential triggers of flare-ups. Identifying triggers can help you avoid them in the future.

- **Rest and Recover:** Allow yourself time to rest and recover when experiencing a setback. Listen to your body and adjust your activities accordingly.

- **Communicate with Your Healthcare Provider:** Notify your healthcare provider about changes in your symptoms or any new challenges. They can provide guidance and adjust your treatment plan if necessary.

- **Stay Hydrated:** Proper hydration is essential for overall health and can help manage symptoms.

MANAGING EMOTIONAL IMPACT

Setbacks and flare-ups can take a toll on emotional well-being. Strategies to manage the emotional impact include:

- Reach Out for Support: Talk to loved ones or join a support group to share your experiences and receive encouragement.
- Practice Stress Management: Techniques such as mindfulness, meditation, and deep breathing exercises can help reduce stress and promote emotional balance.
- Seek Professional Help: If you're struggling with anxiety or depression, consider seeking support from a therapist or counselor.

ADJUSTING TREATMENT PLANS

During setbacks or flare-ups, adjustments to your treatment plan may be necessary:

- Review Medication: Consult with your healthcare provider about potential changes to your medication dosage or type.
- Monitor Thyroid Function: Regular blood tests can help determine if your thyroid hormone levels are stable or need adjustment.
- Consider Additional Treatments: Depending on the severity of your setback, your healthcare provider may recommend additional treatments or therapies.

PREVENTING FUTURE SETBACKS

Taking proactive steps can help prevent future setbacks and flare-ups:

- Maintain a Consistent Routine: Establish a daily routine that includes regular sleep, balanced meals, and physical activity.

- Manage Stress: Incorporate stress-reduction techniques into your routine to help prevent stress-related flare-ups.

- Stay Adherent to Treatment: Follow your prescribed treatment plan consistently and keep up with regular appointments and blood tests.

- Stay Informed: Keep up with the latest research and developments in Hashimoto's management to make informed decisions about your health.

BUILDING RESILIENCE

Resilience is key to coping with setbacks and flare-ups:

- Cultivate a Positive Mindset: Focus on what you can control and practice gratitude for the positives in your life.
- Set Realistic Goals: Break larger goals into smaller, achievable steps to build confidence and maintain motivation.
- Learn from Setbacks: View setbacks as opportunities for growth and learning. Reflect on what you can improve for the future.
- Stay Connected: Maintain strong relationships with supportive friends, family, and healthcare providers.

Conclusion

Coping with setbacks and flare-ups is an essential part of managing Hashimoto's thyroiditis. By understanding potential triggers, implementing coping strategies, and maintaining resilience, you can navigate challenging times more effectively. Stay proactive in your approach to managing your health and well-being, and continue to seek support from your healthcare provider and loved ones when needed.

This chapter discusses strategies for coping with setbacks and flare-ups associated with Hashimoto's thyroiditis, including understanding triggers, managing emotional impact, adjusting treatment plans, and building resilience. Subsequent chapters will continue to provide additional strategies and advice for thriving with Hashimoto's and managing the condition effectively.

CHAPTER 16: NAVIGATING RELATIONSHIPS AND SOCIAL LIFE

Introduction

Hashimoto's thyroiditis can affect various aspects of your relationships and social life, from communication with loved ones to participating in social events. This chapter will explore strategies for navigating relationships and social life while managing the condition. By being proactive and open about your needs, you can maintain healthy relationships and enjoy a fulfilling social life.

COMMUNICATING WITH LOVED ONES

Open and honest communication with loved ones is essential for maintaining healthy relationships:

- Educate Your Loved Ones: Help family and friends understand Hashimoto's thyroiditis and how it affects you. Share information about symptoms and treatment.
- Express Your Needs: Communicate your needs and limitations clearly, whether it's needing rest, adjustments to social plans, or understanding from others.
- Set Boundaries: Establish boundaries to protect your energy and well-being. Be firm but respectful about your limits.

MANAGING SOCIAL ENGAGEMENTS

Participating in social events can be challenging, especially when managing symptoms:

- Plan Ahead: Consider how you will manage energy levels and potential symptoms during social events. Schedule rest periods before and after engagements.

- Choose Suitable Activities: Select social activities that align with your energy levels and interests. Consider smaller gatherings or low-energy activities.

- Keep Communication Open: Let hosts or organizers know about any accommodations you may need, such as seating or breaks during events.

ADDRESSING RELATIONSHIP CHALLENGES

Hashimoto's can pose challenges in relationships, but addressing them openly can help:

- Talk About Your Experiences: Share your experiences and challenges with your partner or close friends to build understanding and empathy.
- Be Honest About Changes: Discuss any changes in mood, energy, or physical health that may affect your relationships.
- Find Solutions Together: Work together to find solutions for any relationship challenges, whether it's scheduling quality time or adjusting expectations.

BUILDING A SUPPORT NETWORK

A strong support network can provide emotional and practical support as you navigate relationships and social life:

- Connect with Others: Seek out support groups, both online and in-person, to connect with others who understand your experiences.

- Involve Family and Friends: Involve loved ones in your journey and lean on them for support when needed.

- Seek Professional Help: Consider working with a therapist or counselor for guidance on relationship challenges or emotional well-being.

NAVIGATING WORK RELATIONSHIPS

Maintaining healthy work relationships is important for overall well-being:

- Communicate with Colleagues: Be open with colleagues about your condition and any accommodations you may need.

- Set Clear Expectations: Communicate your limitations and preferences regarding workload and deadlines.

- Seek Support from HR: If needed, seek guidance from your employer's HR department for workplace accommodations.

BALANCING PERSONAL AND SOCIAL LIFE

Finding balance between personal and social life is key to overall well-being:

- Prioritize Self-Care: Prioritize self-care to manage stress and symptoms. Make time for activities you enjoy and that help you relax.

- Create Social Routines: Establish social routines that work for you, whether it's regular coffee dates or weekend activities.

- Be Selective with Commitments: Choose social commitments that align with your energy levels and interests.

SETTING REALISTIC EXPECTATIONS

Setting realistic expectations for yourself and others can help you navigate relationships and social life:

- Adjust Your Mindset: Understand that some days may be better than others, and that's okay. Be kind to yourself and others.
- Communicate Your Limits: Let others know about your limitations and what you can and cannot do.
- Celebrate Small Wins: Celebrate small achievements and progress in your relationships and social life.

Conclusion

Navigating relationships and social life while managing Hashimoto's thyroiditis requires clear communication, setting boundaries, and building a strong support network. By being proactive and open about your needs, you can maintain healthy relationships and enjoy a fulfilling social life. Continue to seek support and guidance as you navigate these aspects of your life with Hashimoto's.

This chapter discusses strategies for navigating relationships and social life while managing Hashimoto's thyroiditis, including communication with loved ones, managing social engagements, addressing relationship challenges, building a support network, navigating work relationships, and setting realistic expectations. Subsequent chapters will continue to provide additional strategies and advice for thriving with Hashimoto's and managing the condition effectively.

CHAPTER 17: FAMILY PLANNING AND PREGNANCY WITH HASHIMOTO'S

Introduction

Hashimoto's thyroiditis can present unique challenges for individuals considering family planning and pregnancy. Proper management and preparation are essential for ensuring a healthy pregnancy and supporting the well-being of both parent and child. In this chapter, we will explore considerations for family planning and pregnancy with Hashimoto's thyroiditis, including medical management, monitoring, and the postpartum period.

PRECONCEPTION PLANNING

Preparing for pregnancy is essential for individuals with Hashimoto's thyroiditis:

- Consult Your Healthcare Provider: Before attempting to conceive, discuss your plans with your healthcare provider. They can assess your current health status and recommend any necessary adjustments.

- Optimize Thyroid Function: Work with your healthcare provider to optimize your thyroid hormone levels for conception. Proper thyroid function is crucial for a healthy pregnancy.

- Check Nutrient Levels: Ensure your nutrient levels, such as iodine, selenium, and vitamin D, are within optimal ranges for fertility and pregnancy.

- Manage Stress: Incorporate stress-reduction techniques to promote overall well-being during the preconception period.

MANAGING PREGNANCY WITH HASHIMOTO'S

Pregnancy with Hashimoto's requires careful monitoring and management:

- Frequent Thyroid Monitoring: Pregnancy can affect thyroid hormone levels, so regular blood tests are essential to ensure levels remain within the recommended range.

- Adjust Medication as Needed: Medication dosages may need to be adjusted during pregnancy to maintain optimal thyroid function. Work closely with your healthcare provider to monitor and adjust your medication.

- Monitor for Complications: Keep an eye out for potential pregnancy complications, such as preeclampsia or gestational diabetes, which may be more common with Hashimoto's.

- Stay Informed: Educate yourself about the potential impact of Hashimoto's on pregnancy and childbirth to make informed decisions about your care.

SUPPORTING A HEALTHY PREGNANCY

Taking proactive steps can support a healthy pregnancy while managing Hashimoto's:

- Follow a Nutritious Diet: Consume a balanced diet rich in vitamins and minerals to support both your health and the baby's development.
- Stay Hydrated: Proper hydration is crucial during pregnancy for overall health and well-being.
- Prioritize Rest: Rest and sleep are important for managing fatigue and supporting a healthy pregnancy.
- Exercise Safely: Engage in safe, moderate physical activity to promote overall health. Consult with your healthcare provider before starting any exercise routine.

PREPARING FOR CHILDBIRTH

Preparing for childbirth involves considering the potential impact of Hashimoto's on delivery and the postpartum period:

- Discuss Delivery Options: Talk to your healthcare provider about delivery options and any potential challenges related to Hashimoto's.

- Plan for Postpartum Care: Plan for postpartum care, including monitoring thyroid levels and adjusting medication as needed.

- Build a Support System: Enlist the help of a support system, such as family, friends, or a doula, to assist you during childbirth and postpartum recovery.

POSTPARTUM CONSIDERATIONS

The postpartum period can bring unique challenges for individuals with Hashimoto's:

- Monitor Thyroid Levels: Hormonal changes during the postpartum period can affect thyroid function, so regular monitoring is essential.
- Watch for Postpartum Thyroiditis: Be aware of the potential for postpartum thyroiditis, a temporary condition that can cause fluctuations in thyroid hormone levels.
- Prioritize Self-Care: Take care of yourself during the postpartum period by resting, eating well, and seeking support when needed.
- Seek Help for Postpartum Depression: If you experience signs of postpartum depression, seek support from your healthcare provider.

Conclusion

Family planning and pregnancy with Hashimoto's thyroiditis require careful planning, monitoring, and management. By working closely with your healthcare provider and prioritizing your health and well-being, you can support a healthy pregnancy and postpartum period. Continue to educate yourself and seek support as you navigate this important phase of your life with Hashimoto's.

This chapter discusses family planning and pregnancy considerations for individuals with Hashimoto's thyroiditis, including preconception planning, managing pregnancy, supporting a healthy pregnancy, preparing for childbirth, and postpartum considerations. Subsequent chapters will continue to provide additional strategies and advice for thriving with Hashimoto's and managing the condition effectively.

CHAPTER 18: TRAVEL AND ADVENTURE WITH HASHIMOTO'S

Introduction

Travel and adventure can be exciting and rewarding experiences, but they may present unique challenges for individuals managing Hashimoto's thyroiditis. Proper planning and self-care are essential for ensuring an enjoyable and safe trip. In this chapter, we will explore strategies for traveling and adventuring with Hashimoto's, including packing tips, staying healthy while on the go, and adjusting to new environments.

PLANNING YOUR TRIP

Careful planning can help you navigate travel and adventure with Hashimoto's:

- Consult Your Healthcare Provider: Before embarking on a trip, consult your healthcare provider for advice on managing your condition while traveling.

- Plan for Medication Needs: Ensure you have enough medication for the duration of your trip, plus extra in case of unexpected delays. Carry a copy of your prescription.

- Research Your Destination: Learn about healthcare facilities, local customs, and dietary options at your destination.

- Create a Travel Itinerary: Plan your trip with your energy levels and symptoms in mind. Include rest days and downtime as needed.

PACKING ESSENTIALS

Packing thoughtfully can help you stay organized and prepared:

- Medication and Supplements: Pack your medication and supplements in your carry-on bag for easy access. Use a pill organizer for convenience.

- Medical Documentation: Carry a list of your medications, dosage information, and any medical conditions. Include your healthcare provider's contact information.

- Comfort Items: Bring comfort items such as a neck pillow, eye mask, or relaxation tools to help you rest during your journey.

- Healthy Snacks: Pack healthy snacks that meet your dietary needs, such as nuts, seeds, or dried fruit.

STAYING HEALTHY WHILE TRAVELING

Maintaining your health and well-being while traveling is crucial:

- Stay Hydrated: Drink plenty of water, especially during flights or in hot climates.
- Follow a Nutritious Diet: Choose balanced meals and snacks to support your energy levels and overall health.
- Get Adequate Rest: Prioritize sleep and rest to manage fatigue and maintain energy throughout your trip.
- Practice Stress Management: Incorporate stress-reduction techniques such as meditation, deep breathing, or gentle stretching.

ADAPTING TO NEW ENVIRONMENTS

Adjusting to new environments can be challenging, but proactive steps can help:

- Acclimate Gradually: Allow yourself time to acclimate to new climates, altitudes, or time zones.

- Manage Exposure to Allergens: Be aware of potential allergens at your destination and take steps to minimize exposure.

- Monitor Symptoms: Keep track of any changes in your symptoms and adjust your plans accordingly.

NAVIGATING TRAVEL CHALLENGES

Travel can present unexpected challenges, but being prepared can make a difference:

- Carry Emergency Supplies: Pack a small first aid kit with essentials such as bandages, pain relievers, and antihistamines.

- Be Flexible: Be open to adjusting your plans as needed, whether due to weather, transportation delays, or health concerns.

- Seek Medical Help if Needed: Know where to find medical assistance at your destination and seek help if your symptoms worsen.

EMBRACING ADVENTURE SAFELY

Embrace adventure while keeping your health and safety in mind:

• Choose Activities Wisely: Select activities that match your energy levels and interests. Avoid overexertion.

• Listen to Your Body: Pay attention to your body's signals and take breaks when needed.

• Travel with a Companion: Traveling with a companion can provide support and assistance if you encounter challenges.

Conclusion

Travel and adventure with Hashimoto's thyroiditis require thoughtful planning and self-care. By being prepared and proactive, you can enjoy memorable experiences while managing your condition effectively. Continue to seek support and guidance as you navigate travel and adventure with Hashimoto's.

This chapter discusses strategies for traveling and adventuring with Hashimoto's thyroiditis, including planning your trip, packing essentials, staying healthy while traveling, adapting to new environments, navigating travel challenges, and embracing adventure safely. Subsequent chapters will continue to provide additional strategies and advice for thriving with Hashimoto's and managing the condition effectively.

APPENDIX

A: GLOSSARY OF TERMS

- Adrenal Glands: Glands located above the kidneys that produce hormones involved in stress response, metabolism, and immune system function.

- Adrenal Fatigue: A controversial condition characterized by symptoms such as fatigue and difficulty handling stress, possibly linked to impaired adrenal function.

- Adrenaline: A hormone released by the adrenal glands in response to stress, also known as epinephrine.

- Allergy: An immune response to a substance that is usually harmless to most people.

- Antibody: A protein produced by the immune system that recognizes and neutralizes foreign substances.

- Autoimmune: A condition where the body's immune system mistakenly attacks its own cells or tissues.

- Biopsy: A medical procedure in which a small sample of tissue is removed for examination.

- Endocrine System: A network of glands that produce and release hormones to regulate various bodily functions.

- Goiter: An enlarged thyroid gland, often visible as a swelling in the neck.

- Graves' Disease: An autoimmune disorder that leads to overproduction of thyroid hormones (hyperthyroidism).

- Hashimoto's Thyroiditis: An autoimmune condition where the immune system attacks the thyroid gland, causing inflammation and potential hypothyroidism.

- Hormone: A chemical messenger produced by glands in the body that regulates specific functions.

- Hyperthyroidism: A condition in which the thyroid gland produces excessive thyroid hormones.

- Hypothyroidism: A condition where the thyroid gland produces insufficient thyroid hormones.

- Immune System: The body's defense system against pathogens and foreign substances.

- Levothyroxine: A synthetic form of the thyroid hormone T4, commonly prescribed for hypothyroidism.

- Nodule: A small, rounded mass of tissue, such as a growth or lump, that can develop on the thyroid gland.

- Pituitary Gland: A small gland located at the base of the brain that regulates other glands and various body functions, including thyroid activity.

- Radioactive Iodine Treatment: A treatment for hyperthyroidism that involves taking radioactive iodine, which destroys part of the thyroid gland.

- Subclinical Hypothyroidism: A mild form of hypothyroidism with elevated TSH levels and normal T4 levels.

- T3 (Triiodothyronine): One of the two main thyroid hormones, which plays a key role in metabolism and energy regulation.

- T4 (Thyroxine): The primary thyroid hormone, which is converted to T3 in the body to regulate metabolism and energy levels.

- Thyroid: A butterfly-shaped gland located in the neck that produces hormones to regulate metabolism.

- Thyroidectomy: A surgical procedure to remove part or all of the thyroid gland.

- Thyroid Stimulating Hormone (TSH): A hormone produced by the pituitary gland that stimulates the thyroid gland to produce T3 and T4.

B: RECOMMENDED READING AND RESOURCES

- Books:
- "The Thyroid Connection" by Amy Myers, MD
- "Hashimoto's Thyroiditis: Lifestyle Interventions for Finding and Treating the Root Cause" by Izabella Wentz, PharmD, FASCP
- "The Thyroid Diet Revolution" by Mary J. Shomon
- "Why Do I Still Have Thyroid Symptoms?" by Datis Kharrazian, DC, MS
- Websites:
- American Thyroid Association: thyroid.org
- Thyroid Foundation of Canada: thyroid.ca
- Hashimoto's Awareness: hashimotosawareness.org
- The Mayo Clinic: mayoclinic.org
- National Institute of Diabetes and Digestive and Kidney Diseases: niddk.nih.gov
- Endocrine Society: endocrine.org
- Support Groups:
- Hashimoto's Thyroiditis Support Groups: Search online for local or online support groups specifically for individuals with Hashimoto's.
- Autoimmune Support Groups: These groups can provide broader support for individuals managing autoimmune conditions.

- Thyroid Cancer Survivors' Association: A resource for those dealing with thyroid cancer, which may be a consideration for some individuals with Hashimoto's.

C: SAMPLE FOOD DIARY

A food diary can help you track your meals, identify potential triggers, and monitor your nutrient intake. Here's an example format:

- Date: [Date]
- Meal Times: [Record breakfast, lunch, dinner, and snacks with times]
- Meals and Snacks: [Describe what you ate and the portion sizes]
- Symptoms: [Note any symptoms experienced after eating, such as bloating, fatigue, or changes in mood]
- Hydration: [Record water and other fluids consumed, including caffeinated and sugary beverages]
- Nutrient Intake: [Track specific nutrients such as iodine, selenium, and vitamin D, as advised by your healthcare provider]
- Notes: [Include any additional notes about your dietary choices, mood, or other observations]

D: SAMPLE MEDICATION LOG

A medication log can help you track your medication schedule, dosages, and any changes over time. Here's an example format:

- Date: [Date]
- Medication: [Name and dosage of each medication taken]
- Time Taken: [Time of day each medication was taken]
- Notes: [Note any changes in symptoms, side effects, or other observations related to medication use]

E: FREQUENTLY ASKED QUESTIONS

1. Can Hashimoto's be cured?

- Hashimoto's thyroiditis cannot be cured, but it can be managed effectively with medication and lifestyle changes.

2. Can I still lead a normal life with Hashimoto's?

- Yes, with proper management, many individuals with Hashimoto's can lead normal, fulfilling lives.

3. How often should I have my thyroid levels checked?

- It depends on your condition and treatment plan. Typically, thyroid levels are checked every 6-12 weeks when adjusting medication and every 6-12 months once levels are stable.

4. Are there specific dietary changes I should make?

- Some individuals with Hashimoto's benefit from dietary changes, such as reducing gluten, dairy, or processed foods. Consult your healthcare provider before making significant changes.

5. What lifestyle changes can help manage Hashimoto's?

- Lifestyle changes such as stress management, regular exercise, and healthy eating can support overall well-being and thyroid function.

6. How can I find support for living with Hashimoto's?

- Look for local or online support groups, educational resources, and connect with healthcare professionals experienced in managing thyroid conditions.

7. Is exercise safe for individuals with Hashimoto's?

- Yes, moderate exercise can support overall health. Start slowly and listen to your body to avoid overexertion.

F: CONTACT INFORMATION FOR EMERGENCY SITUATIONS

- Primary Healthcare Provider:
- Name: [Name]
- Phone: [Phone number]
- Email: [Email address]
- Endocrinologist (Specialist):
- Name: [Name]
- Phone: [Phone number]
- Email: [Email address]
- Emergency Contact:
- Name: [Name]
- Relationship: [Relationship]
- Phone: [Phone number]
- Email: [Email address]
- Local Hospital/Clinic:
- Name: [Name]
- Address: [Address]
- Phone: [Phone number]

G: SAMPLE BLOOD TEST RESULTS AND INTERPRETATION

Keeping track of your blood test results is important for monitoring your thyroid function and overall health. Here's a sample format:

- Date: [Date of the blood test]
- Test Name: [Name of the blood test, e.g., TSH, T4, T3, or antibody levels]
- Results: [Record the numerical value of the test results]
- Reference Range: [Note the laboratory's reference range for each test]
- Interpretation: [Discuss the results with your healthcare provider to understand their implications]

H: Tips for Communicating with Healthcare Providers

Effective communication with your healthcare providers is key to managing Hashimoto's thyroiditis:

- Prepare Questions: Write down your questions or concerns before your appointment.
- Keep a Symptom Diary: Track your symptoms and share the information with your provider for a more complete picture of your health.

- Ask About Treatment Options: Inquire about available treatments and their potential benefits and side effects.

- Be Honest: Share any changes in your health, medications, or lifestyle to ensure your provider has accurate information.

- Follow Up: Schedule follow-up appointments to monitor your progress and adjust your treatment plan as needed.

I: INTERNATIONAL TRAVEL CONSIDERATIONS

For individuals with Hashimoto's who plan to travel internationally, here are some additional considerations:

- Time Zone Changes: Adjust your medication schedule to account for time zone changes and ensure consistent dosing.
- Language Barriers: Carry a medical alert card or app in the local language describing your condition and medication needs.
- Travel Insurance: Consider purchasing travel

DISCLAIMER

The content of this book, "Surviving Hashimoto's: A Guide to Thriving with Autoimmune Thyroid Disease," is intended for informational purposes only and should not be considered medical advice. It is essential to consult with a qualified healthcare provider for personalized medical guidance, diagnosis, and treatment options.

The information presented in this book is based on research, expert opinions, and the experiences of individuals with Hashimoto's thyroiditis. While every effort has been made to ensure the accuracy and timeliness of the information, new research and developments in the medical field may lead to changes in best practices.

The content of this book was created with the assistance of artificial intelligence (AI). While AI has been utilized to generate and compile the content, it is essential to understand that the information may not reflect the most current medical standards or individual-specific circumstances.

Readers are encouraged to verify any information obtained from this book with credible sources and seek the advice of healthcare professionals for any medical concerns. The authors, publishers, and contributors are not responsible for any adverse effects or consequences resulting from the use or misuse of the information provided in this book.

By reading this book, you acknowledge and accept the terms of this disclaimer and agree to use the information at your own risk.

By including this disclaimer, you inform your readers of the limitations of the content and the role of AI in its creation, as well as emphasizing the importance of consulting healthcare professionals for medical advice.

www.ingramcontent.com/pod-product-compliance
Lightning Source LLC
Chambersburg PA
CBHW052157220526
45471CB00004B/1713